Diet

&

Weight Loss

Explained diet tips and treats thats all you need.

Zunair Ahmad

Contents

Introduction

A significant aspect of good health is a healthy weight. To keep a healthier weight or lose weight, how much you consume and what you eat have a crucial part to play. The other principal-agent is a workout.

For years, low-fat diets were considered to be the best way to reduce weight. An increasing body of research suggests that low-fat diets frequently do not work, in part because these diets often substitute fat with quickly digested carbs.

The perfect weight loss diet is one that is ideal for all aspects of the body, not just for your waistline, from your brain to your fingertips. It is one you will deal with for a long time as well. In other words, A diet that includes a lot of good taste and nutritious options banishes few ingredients and does not require a lengthy and pricey list of food or supplements.

What Is a Diet?

Does the term "diet" cause you automatically think of an awful regime for weight loss?

If that's the case, you certainly wouldn't be alone. For example, in selling food products, consider using the word "diet," which typically defines low-calorie foods, such as beverage diet.

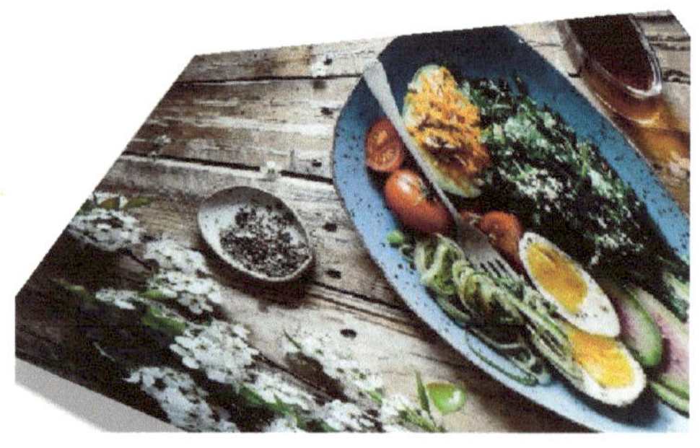

But this word has yet another meaning. Diet may also refer to the drink and food that a person consumes regularly and the emotional and physical problems. Nutrition means more than just eating a "good" diet; it is about food at all stages. Relationships with families, friends, nature (the environment), our bodies, culture, and the world are concerned.

Make Eating A Positive Experience

What and how we eat is sometimes influenced by our feelings and emotions, often in unhelpful ways. Here are some tips on changing lousy diet habits and making our lives a positive feeding experience.

Start Small

Tiny Stage Fruit Don't want to do it all at once. And if you decide what you can do, just choose one thing for a while to adjust and work on that. If it makes you better, add something else.

Listen To Your Body To Recognize And Respect Your Hunger.

Enable yourself to feel the starvation. Accepting it and welcoming it Only be with it for a while and pay attention to what is needed by your body. Don't react to hunger or attempt to remedy it. Anything warm and soothing, or cool and crisp, are you craving? A light or filled thing? Since truly feeling hunger, it is gratifying to feed.

Turn Off The Tv/Screen To Get Rid Of Distractions.

This is highly important. With only the distractions of your head and electronics putting yet another barrier between you and mindful feeding, it is hard enough to stay involved and concentrated on your meal.

Get Involved In Your Diet Before, During, And After Your Dinner.

The crux of mindful nutrition is the option of healthy food. At every point of the meal, think about your food, from the ingredients' growth, to what your body needs, what sorts of textures and tastes you crave, to the pleasure and reflection of cooking it, to sitting down and enjoying it.

Know Your Thoughts, So Do Not Feed Because Of Them.

This is challenging because we experience feelings and control how we feel, which influences what we want to consume and how we want to eat. But when making informed decisions about what to eat, you should consider your thoughts! You're still going to be happy you stopped and behaved purposefully.

Get Rid Of Labels That Are 'Good' And 'Bad.'

There's no reason to beat yourself up or make life more complicated when we learn of diets that are 'good' and 'bad' for us all the time. If you invest resources into taking care of yourself, you deserve sweets and desserts and junk-with no judgment from time to time. You will often find that the cravings shift as you start eating more deliberately, and what was once enjoyable can now be less satisfying and vice versa.

Share Your Food/Your Meal With Others

There are many explanations for eating with others. There is the chance to share the excitement of the food itself and the rare treat of serving others with food that you poured your heart into cooking. There is also such important social encouragement and interaction from friends that sometimes we are more inspired to cook and sit down for a meal when we share it with others or eat them.

Take Your Time

Find out all about being conscious and calming down. This seems to be a specific law, but it's shockingly challenging. We are used to eating on the move, often without stepping out of the car or even slowing down. A significant part of your mindful eating is allowing yourself time all the time you chew to savor your meal and taste each bite. In between bites, bring the fork down. What have you seen? Stop in bites and take a peek at the food on your plate. You become so conscious about your food and practice experience that you don't think about the time.

Stop Until You Feel Full

It is simple to keep feeding because we eat mindlessly and eat without worrying about it. Knowing what it is like to be happy, which is not the same as full, is conscious feeding. It takes about 20 minutes for our brains to get the message that we are full.

There is a point where the appetite is fulfilled, but a small gap may be left, which is a very relaxed and balanced place to be. It is also a means of recognizing and upholding the bounty and privilege we have. Very possibly, more than what we need is what we believe is a normal part.

Enjoy The Process, Have Fun

It's essential to have fun eating. Find out what part you most like in mindful eating and do it more. Is it the food, the gardening, or the table setting? Whatever it is, find ways to integrate it and make it enjoyable into your routine. Be sure to make the schedule part of it. If you want to succeed in eating deliberately, you should enjoy it.

What is Diet planning?

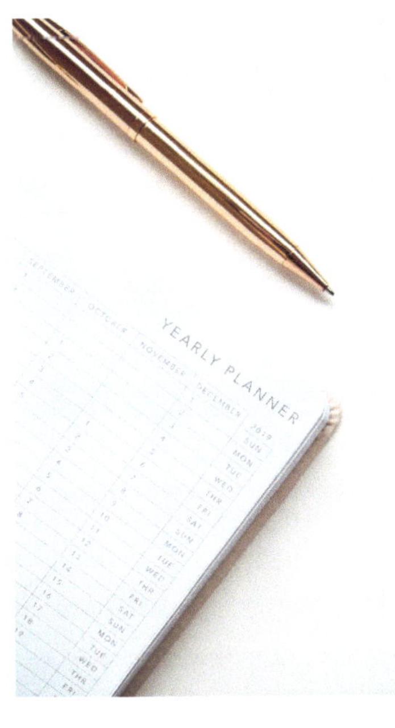

Many individuals equate short-term weight loss and restrictive food consumption with diets. However, a diet plan is customized to the health status, weight, and lifestyle of a person and their weight loss and health objectives.

To direct your eating pattern, exercise, and lifestyle control towards better health and well-being, the diet plan serves as a bespoke guide.

Diet planning for weight loss

Commercial diets also have unbalanced nutritional ingredients that quickly affect weight reduction, but only in the short term.

Depending on what foods you lack in your diet, these dietary imbalances can also cause some adverse health effects.

To hold the weight off, this will result in a loop of yo-yo dieting, and this process will cause you to recover all the weight you have lost, and maybe perhaps more.

A healthy diet, with the correct quantities of various macro and micronutrients, is essential. It contributes to sustainable long-term weight loss and better fitness by having a healthy diet plan.

Principle of Diet Planning

Here are six concepts that we think are important to implement into a diet schedule.

1. Management of sufficient energy, nutrients, activity, and rest stages for optimal health
2. Balancing different food classes and eating foods in the proper proportion
3. To maintain a healthier weight based on the metabolism and activity levels, eat the required amount of calories
4. Focusing on developing a nutrient-dense diet without being high in calories
5. For foods that are richer in fat or sugar, learning how to be moderate
6. Exploring a diverse diet that offers all the required nutrients for good health

Building Your Bespoke Diet Routine For Weight Loss

The way food is metabolized, and food is broken down into essential nutrients is personal to you. Many different variables, including your ethnicity, age, health, and stress, determine how you metabolize food.

Your stomach's health is also highly significant. Specific functional tests will explain how food is metabolized in your body and whether some essential vitamins and minerals are malnourished.

Exercise and diet will also have a different effect on your metabolism. As well as your daily schedule, the type, strength, and length of training are essential factors that influence weight loss and can be incorporated into your personalized diet plan.

To build a strategy tailored for your body to help you control your weight and achieve your fitness goals, we must consider these variables.

7 Days Diet Plans for Weight Loss

Monday

Breakfast:

- 1/2 cup of egg whites scrambled with one tsp of olive oil, one tsp of chopped basil, 1 tsp of grated parmesan, and 1/2 cup of cherry tomatoes
- 1 whole-grain toast slice
- 1/2 a cup of blueberries
- 1 cup of Milk Skim

Snack:

1/2 cup Greek fat-free 1/4 cup of strawberry pieces topped with yogurt.

Lunch:

Salad prepared with 3/4 cup of fried bulgur, four parts of chopped chicken breast, 1 tsp of low-fat shredded cheddar, diced veggies (2 tsp of onion, 1/4 cup of sliced zucchini, 1/2 cup of a bell pepper), 1 tsp of chopped cilantro, and 1 tsp of low-fat vinaigrette

Snack:

2 tspns hummus and 6 carrots for babies

Dinner:

- 4 ounces of salmon grilled
- 1 cup of wild rice with 1 tsp of toasted slivered almonds
- 1 cup of wilted spinach for babies with one tsp of olive oil each, balsamic vinegar, and rubbed parmesan
- 1/2 cup of cantaloupe diced topped with
- 1/2 cup of raspberry all-fruit sorbet and 1 tsp of chopped walnuts

Tuesday

Breakfast:

- 3/4 cup water-prepared steel-cut or old-fashioned oat-meal;
- 1/2 cup of stirred skim milk
- 2 country-style turkey sausage ties
- Blueberries for 1 cup

Snack:

- 1/2 cup ricotta cheese without fat and 1/2 cup of rasp-berries, and 1 tspn of sliced pecans
- 1/2 cup cottage cheese without fat or 1/2 cup salsa

Lunch:Dinner

- 1 burger of turkey
- 3/4 cup of roasted broccoli florets and cauliflower
- 3/4 cup of rice brown
- 1 cup of salad with spinach and 1 tspn of soft balsamic vinaigrette

Wednesday

Breakfast:

- 1 whole egg omelet and Four egg whites
- 1/4 cup of chopped broccoli
- 2 tspns of fat-free refried beans each, sliced onions, diced mushrooms, and salsa
- Quesadilla prepared from 1/2 of a small tortilla of corn and 1 tspn of low-fat fruit cheese
- 1/2 cup of watermelon diced

Snack:

1 chopped apple and 1 tspn chopped walnuts, 1/2 cup fat-free almond yogurt

Lunchtime:

- Salad made of 2 cups of Romaine sliced, 4 ounces of grilled/baked chicken,
- 1/2 cup of celery chopped,
- 1/2 cup of mushrooms diced,
- 2 tspns of low-fat cheddar shredded and 1 tspn of low-fat Caesar dressing
- 1 nectarine medium
- 1 cup of skim/low-fat milk

Snack:

- 1 fat-free stick of mozzarella string cheese
- 1 orange medium

Dinner:

- 4 ounces of barbecued or sauteed shrimp with 1 tspn of olive oil and 1 tspn of chopped garlic
- 1 artichoke medium, steamed

- 2 tspns of diced bell pepper,
- 1/4 cup of garbanzo beans,
- 1 tspn of chopped fresh cilantro
- 1 tspn of fat-free honey mustard dressing,
- 1/2 cup of whole wheat couscous

Thursday
Breakfast:

- 1 light English whole-grain muffin with 1 tspn nut butter and 1 tspn sugar-free spread of fruit
- 1 honeydew wedge
- 1 cup of skim/low-fat milk
- 2 Slices of turkey breast

Snack:

1 cup of low-fat strawberry yogurt, 2 tspns of sliced raspberries or strawberries, and 2 tspns of low-fat granola parfait yogurt

Lunchtime:

- Four ounces of thinly sliced lean roast beef, 1 6-inch tortilla of whole wheat, 1/4 cup of shredded lettuce, 3 long tomato strips, 1 tspn of horseradish, and 1 tspn of Dijon mustard.
- 1 tspn of chopped basil and 1 tspn light Caesar dressing, 1/2 cup of pinto beans or lentils

Snack:

8 chips of baked corn with 2 tspns of guacamole (try 1 of these guac recipes)

Lunch:Dinner:

- Grilled halibut 4 ounces
- Sauteed 1/2 cup of sliced mushrooms with 1 tspn of olive oil, add 1/4 cup of chopped yellow onion and 1 cup of green beans
- Salad prepared with 1 cup of arugula, 1/2 cup of cherry tomato halves, and 1 teaspoon of balsamic vinaigrette
- 1/4 cup fat-free vanilla yogurt, 1/2 cup warm unsweetened applesauce,
- Chopped pecans and 1 tablespoon dash of cinnamon

Friday
Breakfast:

- 1 medium-full wheat tortilla, 4 steamed egg whites, 1 tsp of olive oil, add 1/4 cup of Fat-free crispy black beans, 2 tspns of salsa, 2 tspns of low-fat grated cheddar, and 1 tspn of fresh coriander.
- 1 cup of melon mixed

Snack:

- 3 slices of cooked beef cut
- 1 mid-sized apple

Lunchtime:

- Burger with Turkey (or one of these veggie burgers)
- Salad made with: 1 cup of spinach for babies, add 1/4 cup of cherry tomatoes, with 1/2 cup of cooked lentils, 2 tspns of rubbed parmesan, and 1 tspn of light Russian dressing
- 1 cup of Skim Milk

Snack:

- 1 fat-free stick of mozzarella string cheese
- 1 glass of red grapes

Lunch:Dinner:

- 5 ounces of wild salmon grilled
- 1/2 cup wild or brown rice
- 2 cups of tiny mixed greens with 1 tsp of low-fat dressing for Caesar
- 1/2 cup strawberry sorbet all-fruit with 1 sliced pear

Saturday
Breakfast:

- 3 large egg whites, 2 tspns of sliced bell peppers, 2 tspns of chopped spinach, 2 tspns of part-skim shredded mozzarella and 2 tspns of pesto, 1/2 cup of fresh strawberry/raspberries
- 1 little muffin with bran
- 1 cup of Skim Milk

Snack:

- With 1 tspn Ground walnuts and 1/2 cup of pear diced, 1/2 cup of low-fat nonfat yogurt

Lunchtime:

- 4 ounces breast sliced turkey
- Tomato-cucumber salad with 5 tomato slices, 1/4 cup of chopped cucumber, 1 tspn of freshly chopped thyme, and 1 tspn of Italian dressing without fat
- 1 orange medium

Snack:

3/4 cup of skim milk smoothie, ½ of avocado, 1/2 cup of low-fat cream, and 1/4 cup of sliced raspberry/ strawberries

Lunch: Dinner:

- Baked with 1 tspn of olive oil, 1 tspn of lemon juice, and 1/2 teaspn of no-sodium seasoning, 4 ounces of red snapper
- 1 cup of spaghetti squash, 1 tspn of olive oil, 2 tspns of rubbed Parmesan cheese
- 1 cup green steamed beans with 1 tspn of sliced almonds

Sunday
Breakfast:

- 2 thin slices of beef
- 1 toaster waffle whole-grain with sugar-free fruit spread
- Cup of 3/4 berries
- 1 cup of skim/low-fat milk

Snack:

1/4 cup of cottage cheese without fat with 1/4 cup of cherries and 1 tablespoon of sliced almonds

Lunchtime:

- 2 cups of baby spinach, 4 ounces of grilled chicken, 1 tspn of ground dried cranberries, 3 dices of avocado, 1 tspn of slivered walnuts, and 2 tspns of low-fat vinaigrette salad
- 1 single apple
- 1 cup of Milk Skim

Snack:

- With 1 tsp sugar-free fruit spread and 1 tspn ground flaxseed, 1/4 cup plain fat-free Greek yogurt
- A cup of 1/4 blueberries

Lunch: Dinner:

- Tenderloin of 4 slices of cooked beef stir-fried with broccoli, onions, garlic and bell pepper
- 1/2 cup of rice brown
- Five slices of medium tomato with 1 tspn of chopped ginger

each, light soy sauce, chopped cilantro and rice wine vinegar.

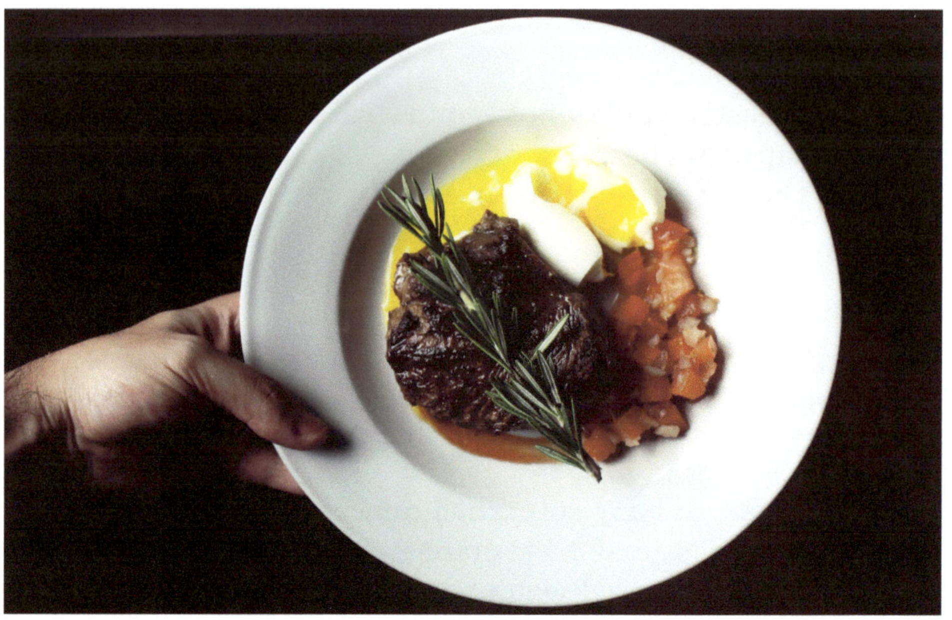

9 tips for weight loss

Here are 9 more tips for a quicker weight loss:

1. Eat a high-quality protein meal. Eating a lot of protein breakfast can reduce cravings and calorie intake during the day.
2. Stop sugary beverages and fruit juices. Empty sugar calories are not beneficial to the body and can discourage weight loss.
3. Drink some water before meals. One research found that before meals, drinking water decreased calorie consumption and could help weight control.
4. Choose weight-loss-friendly food. Any diets are more geared to weight loss than others. Here's a list of safe weight-loss-friendly ingredients.
5. Eat soluble fibers. Studies show that soluble fibers can facilitate weight loss. Fiber supplements such as glucomannan can also help.
6. Drink some coffee or some tea. Consumption of caffeine will improve your metabolism.
7. Focus your diet on all your food. They are cheaper, more filling, and much less likely to induce overeating than processed foods.
8. Feed slowly, man. Eating rapidly will lead to weight gain over time while eating steadily helps you feel fuller and improves weight-reducing hormones.

9. For a decent quality sleep. Sleep is crucial for many reasons, and inadequate sleep is one of the most critical risk factors for weight gain.

Weight loss: 8 techniques for success

Follow these proven methods to reduce your weight and boost your health.

Fast and quick weight loss guarantees hundreds of fad diets, weight-loss schemes, and outright scams. However, a balanced, calorie-controlled diet combined with improved physical exercise remains the cornerstone of effective weight loss. You must make permanent improvements in your nutrition and eating habits for effective, long-term weight loss.

How are you making those permanent changes? Dream of implementing these six weight-loss success strategies.

1. Make Sure You're Ready

Be sure you are ready Long-term weight reduction takes effort, time, and a long-term commitment. If you do not wish to permanently minimize weight loss, you can guarantee that you can make permanent changes to your nutrition and workout habits. To help you assess your readiness, ask yourself these questions:

- Am I motivated to weight loss?
- Am I overwhelmed so much by other pressures?
- Do I use food to deal with depression as a means?
- Am I able to learn to deal with depression or use other strategies?
- Do I need other help to relieve tension, either from friends or professionals?
- Am I prepared to change my eating habits?
- Am I ready to change patterns of activity?
- Do I have the time to invest in making these modifications?

If you need guidance, managing stressors, or feelings that feel like threats to your preparation, speak to your doctor. You'll find it easy to set targets, keep focused, and change patterns when you're ready.

2. Find Your Inner Motivation

No one else will be willing to help you lose weight. To satisfy yourself, you must make diet and fitness improvements. What would give you the raging push to continue your strategy for weight loss?

Create a list of what's important to you, whether it's an upcoming holiday or healthier physical health, to help you stay inspired and focused. Then look for a way to make sure that you will call on your motivational factors during times of temptation. For example, on the pantry door or refrigerator, you may want to post an inspiring message to yourself.

While you have to start taking responsibility for the successful weight loss in your acts, it helps reinforce the right sort. Select people to help you who would inspire you in meaningful ways without guilt, humiliation, or sabotage.

Ideally, locate individuals who listen to your thoughts and emotions, spend time exercising or making nutritious meals, and express the emphasis you have put on developing a balanced lifestyle. Your help group will still have transparency and can be a strong encouragement to adhere to your weight-loss objectives.

If you want to manage your weight loss efforts secret, be responsible to yourself by making daily weigh-ins, logging your diet and fitness success in a diary, or monitoring your progress with digital resources.

Stay Motivated

Permanent weight loss includes the diet and food decisions to create healthy improvements.

To remain motivated/Inspired:

Find a cheering section. Social support implies a great deal. Programs such as Weight Watchers and Jenny Craig use group encouragement to affect lifelong healthy eating and weight loss. To get the motivation you need, seek support, whether in a support group, family, or friends.

Slow but steady to win the race. It will take a toll on your mind and body to drop weight so soon, leaving you to feel tired, exhausted, and sick to lose one to two pounds a week, so instead of water and muscle, you're losing fat.

Set objectives to keep you motivated; Short-term ambitions, such as trying to fit into a summer bikini, typically don't work as well as wanting to feel more secure or to get better for your children's sake. When temptation strikes, concentrate on the benefits of being healthier that you will reap.

Use measures to track your progress. You can keep track of the food you're consuming, the calories you're burning, and the weight you're gaining using mobile applications, health trackers, or simply keeping a diary. You see, the black and white results can help you to stay motivated.

Get lots of sleep. Lack of sleep increases the hunger to get more calories than normal; it stops you from feeling satisfied and making you want to continue to eat. Your motivation can even be influenced by the lack of sleep, so aim for eight hours of quality sleep a night.

3. Set Achievable Objectives

Setting achievable targets for weight loss can sound straightforward. But do you know what's true about that? In the long run, trying to drop 1 to 2 pounds (0.5 to 1 kilogram) a week is wise. In sum, drop 1 or 2 pounds a week, with a reduced-calorie diet and daily physical exercise, you ought to eat between 500 and 1,000 calories more than you need every day. Five percent of your existing weight might be a fair goal, at least for the initial aim., at least for an initial goal, based on your weight. If you weigh 82 kilograms (180 pounds), that's 9 lbs. (4 kilograms). Your risk of severe health conditions, such as heart disease and type 2 diabetes, will be decreased even by this degree of weight loss.

When you set goals, think about the objectives of both processes and results. "Walk every day for 30 minutes" is an instance of a method goal. "Burn 10 pounds" is an instance of an outcome target. You don't need to have an outcome target, but because changing your conduct is the secret to weight reduction, you can set process goals.

4. Cut Carbs

The problem is not consuming too many calories, but rather the way the body accumulates fat after consuming carbohydrates, especially the hormone insulin—a new way to look at weight loss. Dietary carbs enter the body as glucose as you eat a meal. Your body still burns this glucose out until it burns the fat out of a meal to keep the blood sugar levels in order.

If you eat a meal rich in carbs (for example, lots of pasta, rice, bread, or French fries), your body releases insulin to help with the blood flow of all this glucose. Insulin achieves two things in addition to controlling blood sugar levels: it stops the fat cells from releasing fat as a fuel for the body to burn (because its priority is to burn off the glucose). It produces more fat cells to store everything your body can't burn off. The consequence is that you gain weight, and your body needs more fuel to burn now, so you eat more. You crave carbs because insulin only burns carbohydrates, and so a vicious cycle of consuming carbs and gaining weight begins. To lose weight, the logic goes, by decreasing carbohydrates, you need to break this loop.

Most low-carb diets recommend substituting protein and fat for sugars, which may negatively affect long-term health effects. Low-fat dairy goods and lots of leafy green and non-starchy vegetables. In that case, you can reduce the chance and reduce the consumption of saturated and trans fats.

5. Take Note Of Your Food Environment

Build yourself up for success in weight loss by taking good care of your food's environment: when you eat, how much you consume, and what foods you make available.

At home, cook your meals. This causes both food intake and what goes into the food to be monitored. Also, restaurants and processed foods contain much more sugar, unnecessary fat, and calories than home-cooked foods, and portion sizes seem to be more significant.

Serve smaller servings for yourself. To make your portions seem larger, use tiny plates, bowls, and cups. Do not feed on big bowls or food cups directly, making it impossible to determine how much you've consumed.

Eat prematurely. Studies say that it will help you lose more pounds by eating more of your daily calories for breakfast and less for dinner It will jump-start your metabolism, save you from getting hungry throughout the day, and giving you more opportunities to burn your calories by consuming a more extensive, nutritious meal.

Fast For 14 hours a day. Aim to eat dinner late in the day, and then fast until breakfast in the morning. Weight reduction can be improved by eating only when you are most involved and allowing your digestion a long break.

Plan ahead of time for your meals and snacks. In plastic bags or cans, you can make your tiny portions of treats. When you are not hungry, eating on a schedule will help you stop eating.

Drink more water. Thirst will also be mistaken for hunger, so you can prevent excess calories while consuming water.

Limit the amount you have at home of enticing things. Store indulgent foods out of sight when you share a kitchen with non-dieters.

6. Enjoy Healthier Foods

Reducing your total calorie intake must include the adoption of a new eating style that promotes weight loss. But minimizing calories doesn't mean giving up flavor, enjoyment, or even simple preparing of meals.

By consuming more plant-based ingredients, fruits, vegetables, and whole grains, one way, you can decrease your calorie intake is. Strive for diversity without giving up flavor or diet to help you fulfill your objectives.

Get the weight reduction underway with these tips:

- Consume at least four vegetable servings and three fruit servings a day.
- Replace whole grains with refined grains
- Using healthier fats like olive oil, palm oils, avocados, almonds, nut butter, and nut oils in modest quantities.
- Except for raw fruit sugar, cut down on sugar as far as possible.
- Choose low-fat dairy products and small quantities of lean meat and poultry.

7. Get Busy, Remain Active, Stay Active.

Although you can reduce weight without exercising, it can help give you the weight loss advantage with daily physical activity and calorie restriction. Exercise will help you burn excess calories that you can't cut by dieting on your own.

Exercise also has several health advantages, including morale-boosting, digestive system improvement, and blood pressure lowering. To sustain weight loss, fitness will also aid. Studies suggest that those who maintain their weight loss have daily physical exercise over the long run.

How many calories you burn relies on your activities' frequency, duration, and severity. On certain days of the week, one of the easiest ways to shed body fat is by constant physical activity, such as fast cycling, for at least 30 minutes. To lose weight and achieve weight loss, some individuals will require more physical exercise than this.

Any other motion helps burn calories. If you can't get into a day's formal workout, think of opportunities to improve your physical fitness during the day. For eg, take a few trips up and down the stairs instead of using the elevator or, while shopping, park at the far end of the lot.

8. Modify Your Perspective

If you want long-term, effective weight loss, it's not enough to consume nutritious meals and workout for a few weeks or even months. These practices must be a way of life. Changes in lifestyles start with an objective look at the dietary habits and everyday schedule.

While assessing your weight loss issues, aim to build a plan to steadily alter habits and behaviors that have sabotaged your previous attempts. Then move beyond merely recognizing your challenges-planning how to deal with them if you will succeed once and for all in losing weight.

You're probably going to have an occasional setback. But instead of giving up after a loss altogether, just start fresh the next day. Remember that you are planning a life change. It's not going to happen all at once. Stick to your good lifestyle, and it'll be worth the results.

Cheat Days

Diet for 6 days a week, and eat absolutely anything on the seventh. What can't be loved about that? A lot of it. The notion of a "cheat day," or a selected day off a strict diet, stirs up some serious debate in the world of health.

What's A Cheat Day?

In general, there are three views of what constitutes "cheating" on a diet:

Focusing on a particular time frame: the definition that cheating involves eating something over a specified period (one meal, one day, etc.)

Cheating on occasion: for health reasons, eating specific foods you will generally stop, such as fructose to prevent a glucose spike, caffeine to increase stamina, and so on.

Intuitive eating: understanding that cheating is a regular aspect of dieting and is thus not "cheating" at all.

Cheat days can be difficult, but they do bring certain advantages.

Your appetite will dive when you limit calories. To offset any slowdowns, cheat days will help kickstart your metabolism. Splurging will also fulfill the unavoidable urges, allowing you to remain on track for the long term.

Yet cheat days may be the end of yet another weight loss effort.

Here's the reason. The concept of cheating coincides with being on a diet. There is a well-deserved derogatory connotation of the term 'diet.' All is about deprivation. As compared to the new life, you are striving to build, the emotional focus is spent on what you can't get. No wonder the kid in us feels the urge to lie. We want what we want, and right now, we want it!

Let's just play out what comes so much from cheating.

You're floating ahead, pumped, feeling leaner, and energetic about the weight loss. The time has come to rejoice! Join the 'cheat day.' What are you going to want? A juicy cheeseburger with huge fries on the side? A creamy and fluffy cheesecake slice? As much pie for meat-lovers as you can eat? Today is Cheat Day! You should all get them. And because you can, you do.

Then it comes around the next day, and it's time to get back on track. Yesterday's tantalizing flavors are still with you, lingering on your taste buds. With every intention of being "good," you reach the day. But there's no harm in just a tiny bit more. And the downward trend continues, turning a day of cheating into a week of cheating, leading to resentment and surrender.

Then Let's get to the bottom of what's going on.

Your interaction with food is the first problem. You categorize foods as either "good" or "bad." If you eat a bad meal, you're bad, right? You're bad for eating a piece of cake; you're terrible for eating it. You tell yourself, "I really must suck for real." I can't do this. It's silly to believe that I would. Oh, screw it! I'll start again tomorrow.'

Then your childhood is there. Food was a treat for most of us or a punishment. Were you doing your chores? You're having a cupcake! Have you done your homework? It's like chicken fingers and French fries! Haven't you eaten your green beans? For you, no ice cream! Why is it a particular cheat day? The punishment here is a "diet."

Why then are cheat days a good tactic for weight loss?

Since they're done intentionally, they will help the path of weight loss. A couple of years back, but here's the catch: Effectively integrating cheat days into your weight loss strategy requires that you first and foremost have a balanced relationship with food. You must understand that it's your body's oxygen. Not that you can't enjoy it, but you have to be in charge, not the other way around, of that slice of cheesecake.

When you're "on," that is, when you're "good," you have to be 100 percent on, the second crucial aspect of a great cheat day. I've been using lemon juice in my dressing salad. I was particular about the portion sizes. For the six other days of the week, I didn't eat one little nibble of any high-calorie, off-plan food. You're getting the idea.

Then Is a cheat day good for you?

Yeah, but only if the following things can be done:

- keep remorse and negativity Out of the picture.
- Limit your day as a cheat to a day
- After a cheat day, pull yourself right back up and never look back,

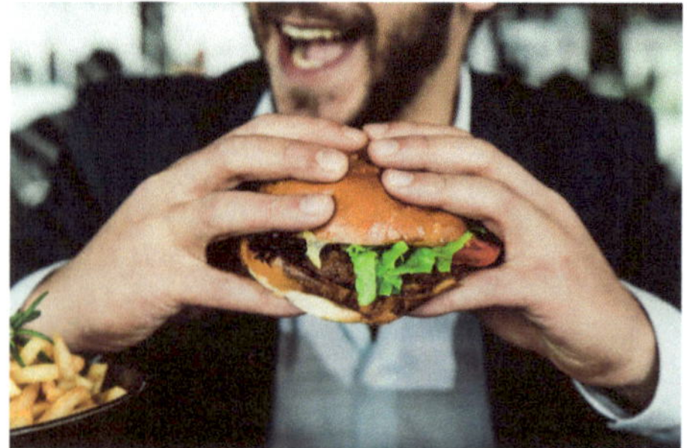

Could you have done that? If not, don't fool yourself or sabotage yourself. Find another approach for you that works.

How Strict Should Your Diet Be?

Are you aware that in the long term, denying yourself of foods you enjoy could destroy your efforts at a fat loss? If you'd like to lose weight permanently and healthily without deprivation, binges, or other food horrors, so here's what you have to do instead.

Find a reasonable way to incorporate all of your ideal foods into your diet, but do it in a manner and frequency that does not sabotage your progress.

This is possible in two ways.
1. Having a regular "free meal" (a.k.a. "cheat meal) is the most common technique." For good reason, you can eat anything you want for this single meal.

2. Another technique most prefer is to work these "treat foods" into your daily calorie allowance, but still make sure that you always get enough protein and healthy fats through your other meals.

It is essential to find balance.

So many meals or days of the program, and the outcomes are compromised. Too many days in a row and you go crazy with cravings, eating nothing but "diet food."

How strict you have to be in your diet schedule ranges from person to individual. That depends a lot on how optimistic your ambitions are and how sensitive your body is to diet and exercise.

Keep in mind that when making your decision, we all have distinct genetics and body types, which is something I discuss in my book, The Flat Abs Formula, in great detail.

For example, are you a carb-tolerant mesomorph that quickly gains muscle and easily loses fat, or are you a carb-sensitive endomorph who quickly gains fat? Your diet schedule can need to be more or less strict than others, depending on the response.

It is advised to consume 90% of the time "on-plan," and 10% of the time "off-plan" food. If you change your enforcement standard above 90% (get stricter) or below 90% (get more lenient) depends on how far or close you are from meeting your targets, and most significantly, what kind of performance you get every week.

If you're 90 percent of the time complying, and you're getting great results, then you don't have to change anything, and you may even be able to loosen your diet a little bit.

90% compliance means that you follow 9 out of 10 meals, or for most of your calories every day, healthy nutritious, fat-burning eating guidelines.

100 percent compliance is unrealistic and unnecessary, even for those fitness models and bodybuilders preparing for competitions. However, option 2 of working favorite foods into calorie and macronutrient limitations would be the way to go in this scenario.

You can do this with absolutely NO set-back to my physique goals as long as you fulfill your minimum protein and healthy fat requirements and remain within your calorie allowance! Moderation and equilibrium are key. Allow some leeway for yourself. Just make sure to keep your calorie caps in mind, and then keep your pledge to yourself and keep to it when you think you're going to hit 90% of the time! Remember: a poor plan is an utter lack of pleasure food since you still want to desire something you can't get. This is a binge waiting to happen. Discover your "healthy equilibrium" and create a sustainable diet and appropriate for your body type.

About The Author

Zunair Ahmad

Zunair Ahmad lives in Leeds, United Kingdom with his wife Miss Muniba Farrukh.

Zunair Ahmad works in a retail and his hobbies are book writing, book reading, online researches for anything ⬚ and he runs his own drop shipping store on Amazon and eBay. Zunair's wife teaches Maths and religion subjects in a school. They've got married in 14/Nov/2014.

Books By This Author

Die, You Damned Robot

Please Remember. This is not an ordinary sci-fi novel, nor a graphic novel.

Ten Years ago, a certain law was passed by the high council that made the very existence of the Megatrons, the most advanced family of robots, illegal. Thus, commencing an era where humans began hunting down their own creations without mercy.

Jun Cason, the protagonist of this world far into the future is sentenced to death for committing one of the worst crimes of recent times. While drowning in depression and awaiting his death, one day a strange man visits him and makes him an offer: spend the last two weeks of your life in this tiny jail cell or live for one week as a free man; only catch is, you'd have to go to that mysterious place in the galaxy where living things die of unknown reasons for our research project. Finding a tiny ray of hope in the darkness, Jun accepts the offer.

On his last day as a free man, Jun witnesses a very cruel public execution of the megatrons while being out on the streets. Megatrons resembles human beings. So, when he sees a teenage megatron girl getting violently killed right in front of him, his sense of justice arises and he ends up saving the girl's lover, a megatron teenager named Nixon. Out of gratitude, Nixon attempts to save Jun from the peril that awaits him in the outer space, but ends in failure.

How could Jun ever hope to survive the Obion planet clusters where the deadly aliens lurk? After learning the conspiracy and the corruption of the high council who rules the world, would he be willing to assist the revolutionaries and help them by committing the same crime that got him a death sentence once again? Follow along as Jun faces one perilous trail after another and rises against the most powerful super computer humanity has ever built, the terrible tyrant Keygen Computer!

Diet & Weight Loss: Explained Diet Tips And Treats Thats All You Need.

This book contains 7 days Weight Loss through out day meals + snacks. An explanation of diet, diet planning, bespoke diet routine for weight loss, 9 use full tips to loose weight, weight loss 8 techniques and cheat days management.

Reviews

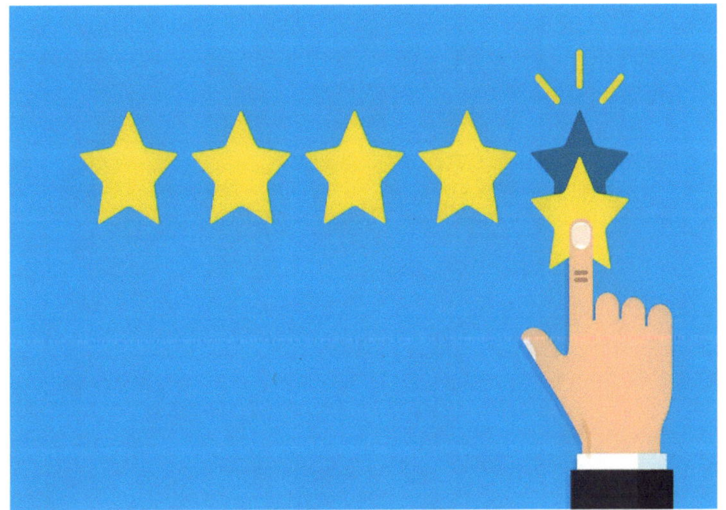

Please submit you reviews by pressing a link below

https://www.amazon.com/dp/B08T1SSXZ2